eBook ISBN: 978-1-7391461-1-5
Paper back: ISBN-13: 978-1-7391461-0-8

Audiobook read by Emma Easton

Cover design by Frank Prendergast
https://www.frankandmarci.com

DOZE AND DIE has been created in American English, utilizing spelling conventions and vocabulary typical of North America.

DOZE AND DIE is available on Kindle, as a paperback and as an audiobook via most online platforms.

Foreword

DOZE AND DIE is a dramatization rooted in real-world evidence and informed by my 30 years of experience in the field of sleep medicine. As the CEO and founder of the British Society of Pharmacy Sleep Services (BSPSS), I have dedicated my career to making sleep expertise accessible.

Sleep disorders not only impact an individual's quality of life but also contribute to a myriad of chronic health problems, including obesity, cardiovascular disease, diabetes, and depression.

As a sleep health advocate, I have also grappled with the ethical dilemmas and systemic barriers that can hinder access to proper diagnosis and treatment.

By weaving together scientific research, sleep expertise, and personal narratives, DOZE AND DIE aims to raise awareness about the importance of sleep health and the transformative power of accessible, evidence-based interventions.

Other than that, I hope you enjoy it!

Adrian Zacher
CEO, British Society of Pharmacy Sleep Services
PhD Researcher, VUB (Vrije Universiteit Brussel).

For Emma, Adam, Elodie,
Nanny and Nellie, the cat.

Important note

This story depicts sleep disorders and medical conditions. If you have concerns about your sleep or health, consult a qualified medical practitioner – ideally a sleep-trained healthcare professional. Do not change your medication without discussing it with your physician first, as this could worsen your condition.

When to seek medical advice

Consult a sleep-trained healthcare professional if you can't sleep, keep falling asleep, or something happens that you don't like when you go to sleep. They can assess your symptoms and recommend appropriate treatment options.

Prioritize your well-being

Poor sleep can significantly impact your health and quality of life. If sleep disturbances interfere with your daily functioning, seek guidance from a healthcare provider specializing in sleep medicine to identify the cause and develop a personalized treatment plan.

Praise for DOZE AND DIE

"Really, very good".

Gareth Evans, President BSPSS.

"Whilst "Doze and die" is a fictional story, it represents many of the real-life issues that so many people with undiagnosed sleep disorders face.
Treatment of a sleep issue can literally save lives.
There's nothing fictional about that!
Congratulations to the author for raising awareness of this vitally important issue!!"

Joanna Kippax, nurse prescriber, sleep practitioner.

"You can clearly picture the families involved, and sadly, the scenarios are very realistic, even though the stories themselves are fiction. Don't shy away from the reallly behind the fiction. If you are recognizing yourself in any of these characters, this is your wake-up call to get help. Great job of bringing the characters to life"

Nicole Ratcliffe, The Workplace Sleep Coach and Family Sleep Specialist

"DOZE AND DIE is a must read for anyone getting behind the wheel of a vehicle because lives can change in the 'slow' blink of an eye..."

Kate Gondouin,
International Wellbeing & Possibility Coach

Prologue

Helen walked smack into the sickly sweet, chemical cloud exhaled from one of several sets of lungs, all sucking like crazy on little plastic sticks with glowing lights.

Pausing for a moment, 'gobby girl' looked at Helen. Scanning her up and down like airport security. Helen wished she'd taken a different route round the school buildings.

"Hey Helen, nice shoes!"

They all burst out laughing, as if it was joke of the year. The cloud of vapor redoubled.

It's like this all the time. Her shoes are awful. It's true. Scuffed and worn. The heel coming off the left one.

And her clothes don't fit. She'd grown and her Mom was struggling to keep up with the bills. Rent, food, utilities and fix the car. Helen didn't want to add to it.

"No, don't go", a kinder tone used. A new, boxed vape is offered. It's brightly colored and looks appealing.

Offered by an arm extended across her only way past them. Sensing blood the pack reconfigured around Helen. Still sucking and puffing.

Helen takes the vape.

Puts down her school bag and takes up vaping.

Just like that.

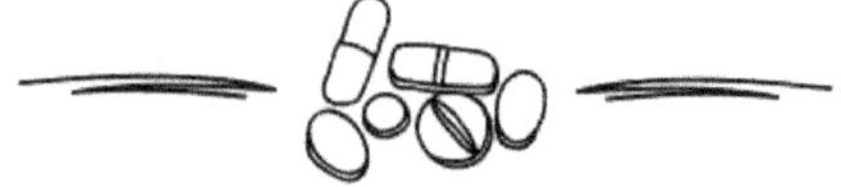

There IS chemistry.

They're both talking too fast and trying desperately not to screw up. The first date ends with a kiss and embrace that grows increasingly passionate. Breaking apart they agree to meet tomorrow. Same place, same time.

There's a certain glow.

Robert and Val. They build a life together, exactly as it's meant to be. They love each other very much and when kids arrive it's hard to believe it can get better.

As the years pass, he begins to snore and at times they 'discuss' it but do nothing about it. Val typically falls asleep before him, so it's rarely mentioned. Ear plugs.

Robert's father had diabetes, so he knows what he should and shouldn't eat but it's become a struggle. He's getting fatter and Val says he's irritable; not the man she married. They discuss it and Robert insists it's work stress and 'getting older'.

The constant fatigue creeps in unseen.

$$_z z^z z \quad _z z^z z \quad _z z^z z$$

"It won't start. Look forget it. Cranking it over and over will just kill the battery". He said to me.

This bloody car is driving me mad. Every time I need to go somewhere, and its important, it refuses to start. It's like it's possessed!

I'm trying to get a job.

So, I reply, "If you know it's broken then why don't you fix it? I mean why leave it until RIGHT NOW - when I need to go for an interview - and now you tell me it doesn't go? Come on!"

Yeah, I'm angry. Pissed off too. I can't keep dodging the bills. Our debt is out of control. Why, when they can see you're struggling with money, do banks whack on charges?!

"So that's another job I won't get", I grumble, climbing out and retrieving my bag from the front passenger footwell.

Resigned I call and get told not to bother when I ask to reschedule.

The truth is we can't afford to repair the car. And I know this. I guess I'm just venting. Oh, by the way, I'm Helen's Mom.

I don't want a sales job. I want to help people. But I've got bills to pay. I used to work in a care home looking after the old folk, but the money's ... well let's be honest, it's not enough.

Back in the house I use my phone (WiFi has been disconnected - don't ask) and search the job sites.

Keep seeing adverts for Panacea Pharma.

They must have a tracking cookie on my phone. But that's stuff I don't know much about.

Look at that basic salary! That would change things. I can't keep 'borrowing' from my parents. And my boyfriend is no help.

I filled in the application form and hit submit with a heavy heart. Working as a drug sales rep.

Someone has to do it, I guess, and this time that someone is gonna be me.

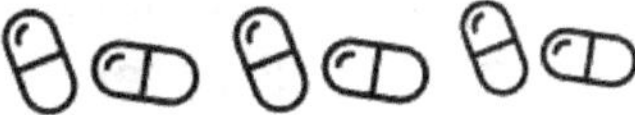

I can almost taste it!

Wash this damn grit out of my throat. I've been thinking about beer the whole tour. And now finally we're almost home. Don't care what time of day or night it is, I'm out and I'm not going to stop drinking until I've had my fill. I've months to make up for.

We'll all go to the nearest and grab a few pints and when it gets too crowded, go into town. Work our way through the bars and back to the nearest one again.

Beer is enough for me. Seen the druggies bent over or collapsed in the street. The Army has zero tolerance for drug use, and I get tested randomly. In Iraq there are enough nutters running around shooting into the air, without them letting me loose with 30 live rounds, stoned out of my head.

But back home on leave, well maybe. Actually, if I'm honest with you not maybe at all. But I don't want that mad stuff. I want OxyRelief. Yeah, you've heard of it. I know exactly what I want and I'm pretty sure where I can get it.

"Move your ass, Troy!" they said before they dropped the pallet on me from the helicopter. We laughed about it at the time and well, when I was home on sick, they put me on OxyRelief for a while.

But I needed to get back out there, so I doubled up the amounts and got going. They thought I'd made a rapid recovery.

I didn't tell them otherwise.

Now, I needed to get some Oxy.

Tonight. Enough for a few weeks if I can get it.

After a few beers.

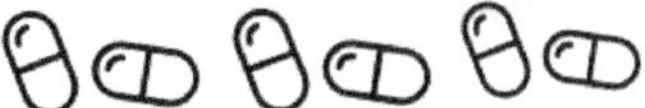

Helen's Mom got the job. She got paid. She got a company car. They sold the old heap and the cash from it bought a pizza that evening.

They gradually caught up with the bills and Mom even talked of booking a summer holiday. As if Helen wanted to holiday with her Mom and new boyfriend!

Helen openly vaped. Her Mom said it wasn't as bad as smoking cigarettes, so while she was disappointed in her, she let it go.

They argued about it. "After all Mom, you sell drugs for a living".

"Oh, but they're prescription drugs darling. For people living with terrible pain".

"Whatever Mom. You know I can buy OxyRelief at school, right?"

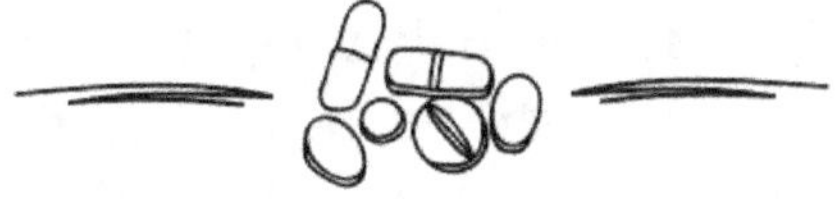

Swerving back to his own side of the road, the paperwork on the passenger seat flying about, he wound down the window and turned the music up loud.

Heart pounding, he was shocked back to alertness.

Robert had dozed off at the wheel.

Again.

He'd be home in a few minutes, and he'd forget all about it; it would be as if it had never happened.

Robert loved his kids. Loved his wife. But he'd never felt so tired. Fatigue was like grappling with a living, breathing animal. And one far stronger than him.

Val had post-natal depression after their first daughter was born and they didn't know at first. Then she was concerned about the antidepressant being present in her breast milk, however small, as she fed the baby. So, despite the physician's reassurance, she wouldn't take any pills.

Now with their second baby, Robert looked after the children at night, so Val could sleep. During the night if his newborn daughter stirred, he'd lie on the sofa and rock the crib that was parallel to it, gently with his foot. The motion soothed the baby and often she'd go back to sleep. For what felt like minutes.

Robert lay there in the small hours struggling to breathe. His chest felt like it wouldn't open. Couldn't get a breath. He knew that if he worried about it, it would only make it worse.

So, he tried to relax. Remain calm. The asthma nurse had given him an inhaler a few weeks ago. It seemed to help at first. Now it did nothing.

He'd forgotten the bit she'd said about it only having 200 doses. It had no counter on it and gas still came out when he used it. But he didn't know it - no medicine.

Robert left for his shift at 03:35hrs so she'd have that disturbance and early morning awakening. And not being a morning person that was not welcome. Robert would be back before 9am and he'd take over 'Daddy duties' when her maternity leave was over. They'd get through. They knew it was tough adjusting their lives to cope with a baby. They'd done it before with their first daughter.

But something was different. Their baby cried and cried. Wouldn't settle. The years went by, and she started nursery. Robert's asthma was now much better controlled, and he could catch up on sleep while both their daughters were out.

'Circadian Rhythm' and 'Shift Work Disorder', please allow me to introduce you to 'Financial Necessity'. And what Robert and Val did not know: ADHD, attention deficit hyperactivity disorder, lurking in the background.

Their little one needed help. They all needed help. And while they didn't know at first to ask, when they eventually did seek help, they were made to feel like failing parents.

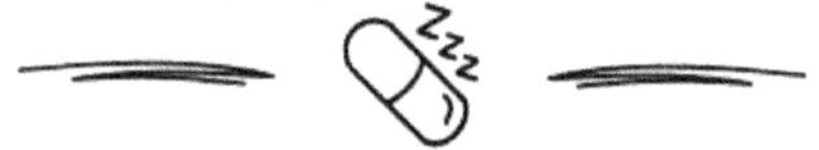

Community pharmacy felt more like a calling than a job. For Ahmed it had always been that way. He'd been brought up caring for others.

Both his parents were pharmacists, and when they began their business, it was just the two of them. They'd taken over the corner pharmacy, and lived in the flat above, because it was close to their families. It was where they had been brought up. It was home.

Gradually they'd modernized the business and planned to get a picking robot when they could afford it. But it was a significant investment. They knew it made sense, and it would save time and reduce errors. Yes, they'd read the leaflets and absorbed the sales message.

Their long opening hours, location and central role within so many people's lives, meant they were part of the very fabric of society.

They were invisible. Yet at the same time essential.

In other words, taken for granted.

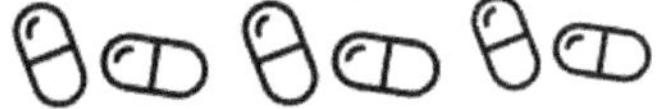

He knew it.

They knew it.

One of those unsaid things: Ahmed was to become a pharmacist.

But before that he had to pass his exams.

While he wanted to be a pharmacist like his parents, it sometimes felt like an obligation.

It was expected of him.

The pressure mounted and fueled his insomnia.

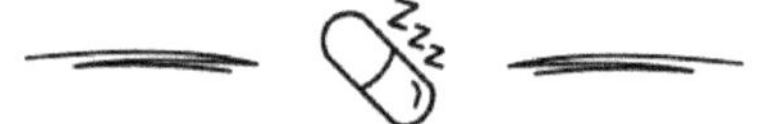

OxyRelief.

Again, thought Ahmed's dad. He was definitely seeing more prescriptions for it. "It's an opioid that they say doesn't make people dependent on it", he mused. He was not so sure. Along with more prescriptions he had observed increased dosages. For the same people.

Chronic pain is of course persistent. So maybe that was why. The regulators know what they're doing, so perhaps I'm worrying unduly, he thought.

He moved on to the next prescription.

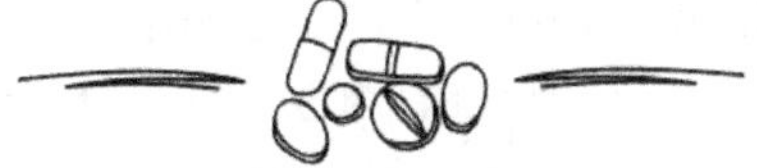

"What age is this for? My daughter is three and really struggling with sleep" Robert asked Ahmed's father, discussing melatonin gummies.

"I'm sorry to hear that, Robert. No, sorry the evidence does not support their use for your daughter's age. I understand they're doing long-term studies on it though. I think speaking to your physician about sleep would be best". The conversation continued around sleep hygiene and behavioral approaches.

Robert explained he and Val were getting little sleep. As their daughter was exhausting. As he discussed it, he felt himself welling up, because it was so good to have someone listen to him.

Regaining control of his emotions, Robert vowed to contact his physician and left.

Ahmed's dad went back to checking prescriptions. Ten minutes here. Five minutes there. Nearly lunchtime already?! Where did the day go? The pile of prescriptions continued to grow.

"We need some help", he said to his wife. Ahmed had always helped after school and on a Saturday. As a kid he began with making coffee and emptying the bins. Moving bulk containers and just trying to help out, pushing the broom round. There were a million little jobs to do that didn't need you to be qualified.

As he progressed through school and then university, he naturally took on more roles.

Ahmed always studied in bed. His bed was where he read, where he revised, where he did assignments. He had to move the books aside to find his pillow and rest his head.

Each night after dozing off in front of the TV, Ahmed went to bed and tried to sleep. As usual he'd be 'ping' wide awake. Which made him try harder to go to sleep.

The corner of the textbook under his pillow, jabbed him in the cheek, as he rolled left and right trying to find a cooler part of his pillow.

He wanted to escape the pressure. He couldn't screw up. Felt his parents would disown him.

Mind racing, worrying about how tired he'd be tomorrow if he didn't sleep, Ahmed was like a dog with a bone, kept pushing himself to 'go to sleep'. As if he could just turn on sleep.

Giving up trying, he stumbled to the bathroom. Another day beginning, he'd grab a few energy drinks on the way in, to stay awake in class.

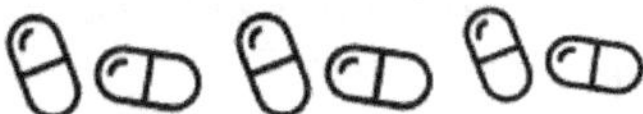

"I need you to help out more. In the morning Robert, I know you're tired when you get back from work, but it's too much to get them both sorted for school on my own".

"Should you be eating that?" Val exclaimed.

His look of disgust the reply.

Robert's diabetes was something he'd expected to develop. His father had diabetes so he knew what he was eating would make his blood sugar spike. Because Val was right, it only made it worse. Made him more resolved to eat it anyway.

Val cared. But the strains in their relationship were beginning to show. Cracks appearing.

They bickered. He snored. She was annoying. He hogged the remote control. She squeezed the toothpaste tube in the middle. He didn't earn enough. All stuff indicative of their lack of sleep.

"I wish you wouldn't moan so much…" Robert finally volunteered. He usually tried the strong, silent routine. Slamming the dishwasher door shut, turning to look at their eldest he said "She will hate you when she grows up. You bully her."

And they were off. Into a full-blown argument about their different approaches to parental discipline.

Tears formed in Connie's eyes as her lower lip quivered. Her parents were shouting at each other again.

Part One

Chapter One

It's called a 'thousand-yard stare' in the military. It's that paradoxical horizon scanning yet seemingly blind, blank look in the eyes. I couldn't see it when I looked at my oppo. Not knowing my own eyes were exactly the same.

Don't run.

I was told that if you ran you could just as easily run to where the next mortar bomb would fall and explode.

So, here I am in my tent, listening to the explosions all around. Wondering if the next one has my name on it. Dread and unspeakable fear fill me up inside as I replay the living nightmares of the previous weeks.

This is my second tour. Three months in Iraq and now I'm in Afghanistan.

My name is Troy, and one day I won't be in the Army.

One day. If I live through this night.

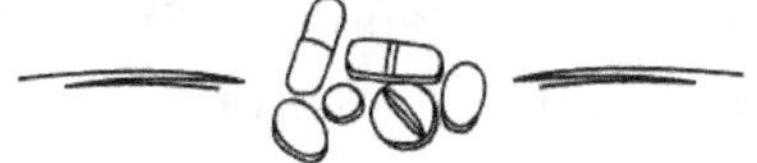

"Turn the bloody music down".

Says the ignored neighbor as they pound on the front door. The bass beat of the music makes the house pulse with a heartbeat.

The party started after the bars shut and by 2am most are in a stupor induced by whatever substance they can get their hands on. The neighbors are of zero consequence. No one sleeps tonight.

In one room the student dropouts hang out, while in the kitchen the nerds and socially awkward, pretend to listen to the music bouncing about inside their skulls.

"Great party", said 'Greasy' to her breasts.

Sarah, sighing inwardly hoped he would disappear, and she could get closer to the man near the door.

She'd come to the party with a new boyfriend and was pretty sure he was upstairs with someone else. She wasn't cool about it but feels she has to pretend to be.

She feels dirty and used. He says she's nothing. Fat and worthless. But the man near the door has something about him. Something indefinable. She doesn't know it yet, but it's because he's dangerous.

And she is messed up. There is something bad there and she is drawn like a moth to a flame.

"It's so lame", he shouts above the music. She nods earnestly as she catches his eye. As if she has the first idea what he's referring to.

Sarah follows him outside where they can at least hear their own thoughts. He says his name is Gary, and she Mombles 'Sarah' several times as he can't hear her above the music. She blushes like a child as he looks at her.

Upstairs, surrounded by a haze of blue smoke, Helen passes the joint back to 'bro'. They've known each other a lifetime of five minutes and said a handful of deep, unheard words.

Fast forward two weeks and Sarah's latest relationship is over. Except now she feels worse about herself. Their contemptuous words engraved in her mind.

Fat. And others not worth repeating.

Self-esteem is a lovely concept - if you have any.

Sarah crashes into her first bout of depression. The student counsellor refers her to the physician, who drones on about what should be but isn't available for five minutes; finally handing her a prescription for antidepressants.

Somehow, the soulless automaton that was Sarah graduates.

The weight piles on.

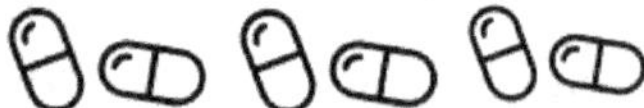

03:35hrs. Tossing and turning he runs through it all again. Ahmed can't sleep. Exams in the morning, and he's worried that unless he gets a good night's sleep he won't pass. It's his weakest topic; it just doesn't stay in his head. Arghh!

Finally, he falls asleep, and after what feels like minutes, his phone alarm wakes him.

"I feel like I've been run over", he groans as he drags himself to the bathroom.

Despite his insomnia, Ahmed graduates as a pharmacist. He is driven to succeed, with a vision of his own pharmacy, serving the community he grew up in.

He's going to make it real. Just you see.

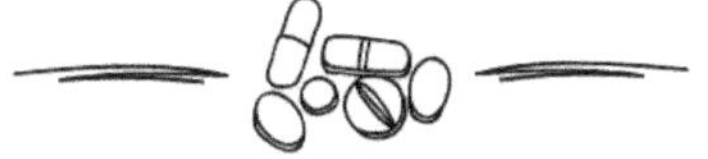

"GO, GO, GOOoo!" So, I leap up and charge in scanning fast. Left, right, up, down.

"Clear!"

Boots stomp past me as we roar through the building. I'm glad to lean against the wall, panting hard, my back absolute murder. Hell, I've done something to it, but right now I CAN move, so I do.

Later, my back seized up bad. 'Brufen' (Ibuprofen) which I've been taking like M&Ms, isn't cutting it.

"Troy, I think you've crushed some vertebrae", the medic said.

I don't give a damn. I've got a job to do and my mates to look after.

Tramadol. That just takes the edge off it.

Hell, what I'd do for a beer... or three.

Keep 'em coming.

Chapter Two

Sarah bit the chocolate. Her headache threatening to split her skull in two.

She knew she was fat. Didn't need the physician telling her she was "obese". They just sat there with a condescending look on their face. Sod them.

"Damn my throat's sore", she thought as she levered herself off the toilet, side-stepped the bathroom scales and struggled into her clothes. Stomach rumbling, feeling dead-tired, fighting back a sick feeling, Sarah trundled off to work.

As she drove, she paused to let some 'crazies' out running, cross the road ahead of her. Getting all hot and sweaty. "What the hell time of day did they get up?"

The day was sure to blend into the usual pattern of feeling tired and hungry. "Well at least I don't have wrinkles" she thought glancing at the rearview mirror. Her headache, nausea and fatigue made her eyes droop at the usual point on her route.

When she woke, her face stinging, she didn't recognize her surroundings, bright lights, something beeping, and scuffling of feet and muffled conversations along the corridor.

 "Where am I?" Quickly replaced with "Why am I in hospital – my boss is going to be pissed if I'm late again".

"You've had an accident", said the white coat next to her. Their words blurring together as she felt her face. Burned by the airbag.

"I'm afraid the police want to have a word with you".

That caught her attention.

"Why?" She asked white coat. "They think you fell asleep and I'm sorry to have to tell you someone died at the scene".

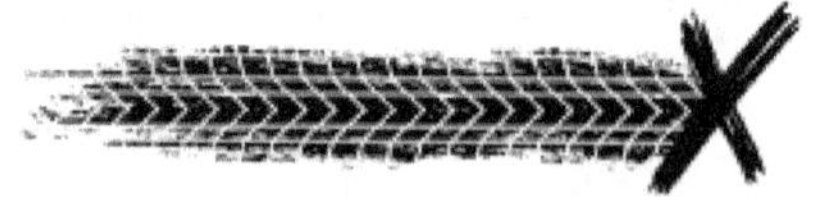

"Oh, that's not fair. I want Sarah in MY team!"

Sarah hadn't always been fat.

As a kid, she was good at sports. Not earth shatteringly so, but respectable. As a young woman, the weight came with the let-down. Every time someone hurt her, she'd comfort eat. Turn towards the Ben and Jerry's. The packets of biscuits. The chocolate bars.

When the weight led to self-loathing, she comfort ate her way through that. It went properly wrong when after a year of 'working at it' she found her husband was still seeing the 'other woman'. Divorce and 'life gets in the way' meant exercise became a thing of the past.

When she couldn't get out of bed on the third morning, her sister marched her to the physician. After a month or so of 'happy pills' and 'group therapy' that left her cold, she sort of resurfaced.

Friends rallied round and a few one-night stands meant some people found her attractive - even if she didn't. Her work ethic kicked in to pay the bills. While her office job gave her structure. It wasn't hard. She showed up each day to the grey building, on the industrial park, argued with the men over the air conditioning thermostat and didn't take work home.

Insomnia was never a problem. When her head hit the pillow, she was out like a light. Dragging herself out of bed each morning was another issue.

Troy was good company at work. He was clearly unhappy with his homelife, and she was alone. They flirted and the banter made her half smile. Which made Troy try even harder. The days blended together.

'Same shit, different day', had become her motto. She was in a rut but couldn't see a way out of it. Didn't even recognize the rut for what it was.

Battling depression, she wasn't going anywhere fast in life.

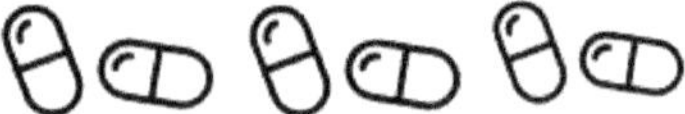

"Damn, these stairs get steeper every day", Troy puffed as he put one leaden leg in front of the other, the pain in his chest growing. "I know I should use the stairs", Ahmed the pharmacist said to keep up his exercise.

"I reckon Ada put him up to that", Ahmed says exercise is important as he knows Troy has high blood pressure.

"To hell with that - it's gonna be the lift after lunch".
The fast-food restaurant had a special running this
week.

Rubbing his tired eyes, Troy plodded on up, wondering
how it got to the point where Ada routinely slept in
another room. "Stop snoring", she complained as the
words disintegrate into the usual shouting match. As if
he chose to snore, just to bloody annoy her!

Ada bought him various things to stop him snoring,
that they sold in the pharmacy. This gadget and that
spray.

He'd tried, honestly, he had. But nothing worked.

He either didn't fit the gadget or they just plain hurt.
Maybe the only way they were intended to stop him
snoring was by keeping him awake! "What a waste of
money. I bet Ahmed made a tidy profit from selling
that rubbish". "Why didn't she just get some sodding
ear plugs?"

Enough already dammit. She'd even said he stopped
breathing in between snores and "She couldn't bear
lying there hoping he would start breathing again".
Whatever!

If she cared, she wouldn't sleep in the spare room.

The door exploded open ahead of him as Robert barged past and charged down the stairs three steps at a time. "Not now Troy. It's Val", he shouted, "She's been in an accident".

Troy doesn't know how lucky he is.

Troy had struggled with sleep for as long as he could remember. He'd describe himself as a 'light sleeper' while his wife Ada would disagree. If she was allowed to have an opinion.

With Troy it was his way or the highway. He liked to think he was reasonable. But he was in reality intractable. Stubborn to put it mildly. Unless it was his physician talking, nobody could tell him anything. Ada had given up arguing with him. Said he had changed. He was always grumpy these days.

"Damn, love – look in the mirror!"

The trouble was, his physician while trying hard to manage his high blood pressure, "not more pills?", never asked him about his sleep. So, Troy never mentioned it. Troy's snoring was Ada's problem, and not his.

Feeling tired all the time was just a fact of life. "Goes with the territory. I work hard and I'm getting older".

"If only I could shift the weight", he thought lifting his gut with both hands where it bulged over his trousers.

He'd tried dieting in fits and starts but he enjoyed his food, considered himself a wine connoisseur of sorts, and without truly realizing it, drank "just a few glasses" every night.

The alcohol and the sleeping pills helped him get off to sleep and he'd grown used to the multiple nighttime awakenings to pee and the morning fogginess.

The physician said to only take the sleeping pills when absolutely necessary. "When aren't they absolutely bloody 'necessary'?" he'd scoffed.

As a young man he'd smoked. Everybody did back then. Now, he viewed the vaping craze amongst the 'youngsters' with jaded eyes. "It's gonna bite you", he'd wheeze to himself.

He wondered idly what had happened to Robert's wife Val. He didn't really know her that well. Seen her at office "Do's" and she was nice enough.

Robert's two little girls were great though. Cheeky, smiley, happy. As little girls should be. Everybody loved them at the summer BBQ, running around giggling. Stuffing cake in with both hands, chocolate smeared across their faces.

"Hope Val's OK. I'm sure it's nothing".

"Better get on with the deliveries. They won't drive themselves" he thought.

Troy was warehouse man and local delivery guy. He considered he knew the business and its customers inside out. Prided himself on it.

"I should be running this place", he said to anyone who'd listen, putting the kettle on to make a big coffee, to take with him in the truck.

First drop the local school. They get through a lot of paper.

Chapter Three

The robot doesn't sleep.

Instead, it whirs mesmerizingly back and forth as another busy day in the community pharmacy begins.

"Morning Ada", greets Ahmed the pharmacist as he arrives, mentally bracing himself, for people querying his 'stupid questions' and complaining about waiting for their medicine.

He didn't sleep well last night. He struggled to get off to sleep and woke very early worrying about keeping his business afloat and being there for his customers.

Some customers they know as friends. And Ahmed is proud to have Ada 'out front' as she always has a smile and kind word. Ahmed begins checking the prescriptions and medicines that are waiting for him. Sipping his coffee, he half listens to Ada and smiles to himself.

"Good morning Troy", smiles Ada. The usual brief chitchat ensues as Ada shuffles back and forth twittering away, looking for Troy's blood pressure and sleeping pills among the alphabetized boxes.

Ahmed glances up, looks over the dividing half wall and notices the dark bags under Troy's eyes. "He doesn't look well. He has the same tired eyes I do", Ahmed doesn't think much about sleep disorders. They weren't part of his university education. He's seen the odd article about sleeping pills or 'Z drugs' and he's done some manufacturer 'training' about insomnia but he's skeptical about how impartial it was.

Yet, he doesn't know how to help Troy or himself for that matter. He knows in general he's seeing more prescriptions for sleeping pills, but he never thinks that much about it.

"It's only sleep after all".

"We've more to worry about" Ahmed muses. "We've an obesity epidemic; a diabetes epidemic and it seems everyone has either high blood pressure like Troy, or depression like Sarah".

He can hear Ada and Troy chatting and overhears "Did you hear Sarah fell asleep at the wheel and killed Val? Can't believe it...".

A storm is building.

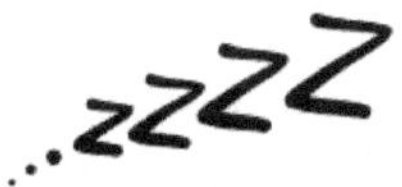

Ahmed runs his hand through his thinning hair, "Poor old Robert. And what about the girls?", he wonders.

When Ahmed was at university, pharmacy was pharmacy he thought. He knew what he was going to be doing. It was about medication. What he didn't know about medicine and interaction between medicines, wasn't worth knowing.

But now he was to come out from the back room, checking prescriptions, to talk with people. Some days that was good. Some not so. He was busy enough as it was and talking to people, while it was great to use his knowledge, took time away from his family.

He routinely ran late into the evening.
It was on him as Superintendent Pharmacist to check the prescriptions. Some things are hard to delegate in a small community pharmacy.

His wife was mostly understanding. But there are limits. Ahmed needed to show up at home, but she knew he couldn't just walk away. Leave prescriptions incomplete. People needed their medicine. So, they argued. Not often, but it was a simmering tension that soured their relationship.

"We need a holiday", thought Ahmed. "But locums get paid more than I do! So, not only do I pay for the holiday, I lose money covering the scheduled hours".

The economic woes of community pharmacy and the cost-of-living crisis meant some of his competitors had already gone out of business. He was busier than ever, but the bottom line didn't reflect that.

"Oh hell. I've got to do my revalidation again; a year's gone so fast". He had some records but needed another Planned Activity.

"And I bet I've gotta pay for that as well…" he grumbled to himself.

"Oh Sarah, what have you done? Should I have spotted her issues? Those poor little girls".

The picking robot continued whirring back and forth.

Unthinking.

Chapter Four

"No Connie you can't take your teddy bear to school.... Isla, I don't know what you do with your hair bands. Go and look for one. A black one not pink".

The usual morning chaos, trying to get the kids out the door, looking halfway presentable. Finally, Val and daughters depart. Holding hands and chattering away gaily about heaven knows what.

Isla and her little sister Connie love school. And when it's dry, they all enjoy walking together to primary school. Today, they chat about going to the park after school. It should be a warm and sunny afternoon.

Maybe, just maybe, Mom will buy ice-cream if they're good.

Connie helps her teacher hand out the spelling tests to the class. The teacher hearing the impact of the car on the school wall and railings, not appreciating the lack of screeching tires, heard just a double thud.

She automatically pulls her class's attention to herself, while drawing the blinds across the window, shielding her class. She sees others rushing towards the car and her focus returns to start the spelling test.

As Connie hands out the test sheets, Isla is daydreaming about ice cream and Mom pushing them on the swings.

The sirens begin to wail in the distance.

At the scene of the crash outside the school, a passerby calls an ambulance while peering in through the side window of Sarah's car. She's out cold.

Fortunately, the engine cut out on impact. He can't get the door open. The emergency services keep the passerby on the phone, as more people arrive and what seems like hours later but isn't, the scene is secured with yards of yellow tape fluttering in the breeze.

Screens go up to hide the motionless body of Val, while photos are taken from every conceivable angle.

There are no skid marks on the road...

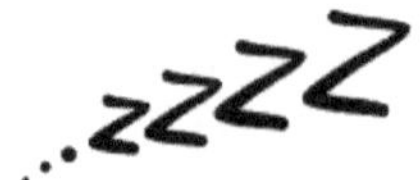

The crime scene investigator looks for Val's ID and as they do so Val's phone rings. Again, and again. The phone is passed to the police officer, who cautiously answers the incessantly ringing phone.

They need to ID the body.

Before the police officer can speak:

"Where are you love? How long does it take to walk back you lazy bum?!"

Tears, disbelief, and anguish.

Soon the sister arrives at the scene. You couldn't keep her away if you tried.

Enroute the sister calls Robert. "She's been hit by a car. See you at the hospital. No, the girls are fine. She was walking back from dropping them off. Look, I've gotta go. Talking to the police".

The police want to talk to Sarah but she's unconscious. The firefighters cut the car door off.

The paramedics take Sarah, now wearing a neck collar, to hospital.

Playtime at the school is delayed. It's difficult for the teachers to stop the kids, Isla and Connie amongst them, from peeking out from behind the blinds, with so much noise and lots of flashing lights right outside the school.

The nervous sister and police officer converse.

"Where's Val?" the sister asks.

The police officer alone knows Val is lying dead on the ground behind the screens. She's called for backup.

It's going to be a long day.

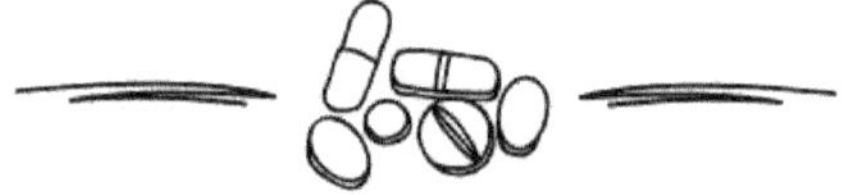

"Why the hell is my sister-in-law calling me at work for God's sake?" Robert grumbles as he puts down his third (or was it his fourth?) cup of coffee of the morning. It's not yet 9am.

And then his world shrinks, goes cold and very dark.

"She's been hit by a car... See you at the hospital... No, the girls are fine...".

Barely hearing the words, Robert strides across the office, forgetting his coffee. Shoves the phone in his pocket as he slams open the door, almost colliding with Troy laboring up the stairs. "Not now Troy", he shouts. "It's Val. She's been in an accident".

Robert, rushing around had missed breakfast, trying to help Val get the kids out the door. At the time he'd chosen get to work a little early rather than eat and be late. With caffeine and adrenaline surging through his body, Robert had to prevent himself, from speeding all the way to the hospital.

Struggling to balance conflicting desires of speeding and risking the lives of others, versus not being around for his kids. Little did he know, that should he crash and die, his girls Isla and Connie, would be orphans and either his sister-in-law would suddenly have a larger family, or they would be taken into care.

The weight of his fatigue temporarily pushed aside with the immediate urgency of the situation; he arrives flustered at the Emergency Room. "Why are there so many police here?" he wonders.

He's asked for ID. Taken to a quiet side room, then asked to identify "the body".

His worse fears are confirmed. She's dead. How can it be?

Numb. Everything a blur.

Silence in his head yet its deafening at the same time. He sees everything and nothing.

Val's sister arrives and manages to force her way through the scrum of blue scrubs and police uniforms, to get to him. They hug. They cry. Trying to hold each other up. He knows he must be there for his kids. Where does he even begin?

How is he going to tell them Mommy isn't coming home tonight? Grief and fatigue hit him like he's run into a wall. The caffeine has run out. But he realizes he needs his meds from the pharmacy.

Looking at the clock above the nurses' station, he estimates he has just enough time to get to the pharmacy then pick up the girls.

He has to be there.

There won't be ice-cream at the park tonight, for two little girls.

Chapter Five

"I've a few questions for you" the police officer says after scaring the life out of Sarah, reading her rights, while she lay in the hospital bed.

"What the hell?!", thinks Sarah, as scenes from TV cop shows race through her mind. This can't be real. Had she really killed someone? "I didn't mean for this to happen".

Disbelief and horror at what they say she's done. "Stop now, I want to get off", she thinks.

The brief interview comes to a blessed end, with Sarah and the police officer agreeing to talk in the morning. She dissolves into tears when he's gone. Rubbing her sore shoulder, bruised by the seat belt and wracked with guilt, Sarah can't hold a thought. She literally doesn't know what to do with herself.

She's discharged and on autopilot finds her way to the pharmacy.

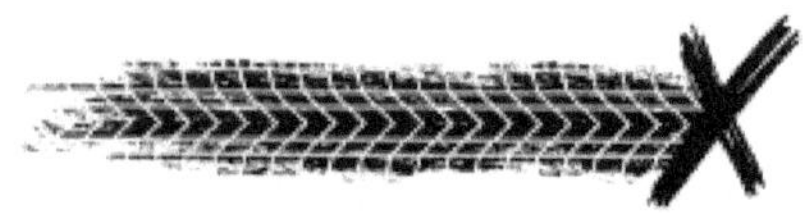

"Hello Robert. How're you?"

"Sorry Ada don't wanna talk. Come to get me pills", as the lump in his throat near chokes him, not even half aware of the large woman behind him in the queue. Tears misting his vision, Robert is shepherded into the consulting room.

Ahmed, the pharmacist gently closes the door behind him.

"What's happened Robert?" Ahmed's usual friendly face marred by a concerned frown.

"It's Val. She's dead. Don't believe it. Can't get me head round it". Robert blurts, tears forming in the corner of his eyes.

"She'd just dropped kids off when car hit her. Don't make no sense..." Ahmed pictures Val and their two daughters, Isla and Connie.

A tap on the door and Ada's head appears. "Ahmed, sorry to interrupt but can you sign this?" she proffers a small plastic box and prescription.

"Well better be off", Robert murmurs through the tissue as Ahmed squiggles his signature while glancing at Sarah's prescription.

Ada takes payment from Sarah for her "happy pills", both of them too polite to discuss what they've seen and the rumor about Val.

Ahmed, turning back, "Sit down please Robert. You don't look good. Lean against the wall Robertl I've got you". The tempo of his voice rising. Robert, his head spinning, with stars in his vision, is lowered by Ahmed back to the chair and he slumps against the wall.

Ahmed regaining control calmly calls Ada back "Ambulance", he urges as he wraps the blood pressure cuff around Robert's upper arm.

Sarah waits outside for an Uber. Seemingly in a trance.

Ahmed records Robert's vital signs as he drifts in and out of consciousness. When Robert wakes up in the Emergency Room, his heart sinks once more as he remembers Val isn't far away, laying cold and very dead in the morgue.

"What about me girls?" he asks of no one.

His mind racing as he tries to sit up. Gentle yet firm hands press him back to the bed. "We think you had a hypoglycemic blackout, Robert. Rest now. Do you have someone we should call? Social services have been informed".

Robert says about Val's sister.

His blood sugar had fallen like a stone. Eating had been far from his mind.

He was a widower and single parent now.

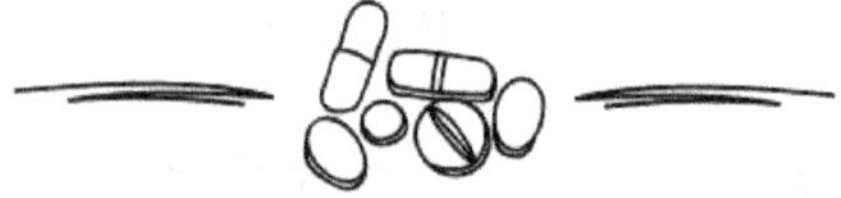

"For short-term use only".

Ahmed wonders what that even means as he hands another customer their OTC[1] 'sleep aid'. He's seen the same customers request the same thing week in and week out.

But what are the alternatives? He doesn't know about Cognitive Behavioral Therapy for Insomnia or CBT-I. He

---

[1] OTC = Over-The-Counter. Meaning available without a prescription.

suggests they visit their physician. Pretty sure he's wasting his breath as they don't take sleep seriously.

"If I don't sell it, they will just buy it elsewhere", he argues with himself. And besides, "What else is there?"

He self-medicates his own insomnia. He is 'tired but wired' and increasingly short-tempered. "What a week?! Val dead, because Sarah is rumored to have fallen asleep, and Robert collapsing".

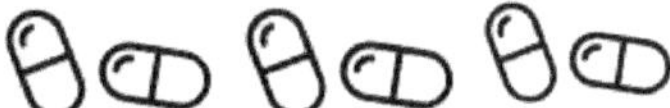

The other side of town, Troy is struggling with what feels like a vice around his chest. He'd stopped at the traffic lights and frustrated drivers pulled out from behind to overtake, swearing and shaking their fists.

He doesn't even register them. "It will pass", he says to himself fighting off the pain, trying to catch a breath. "I'll get some indigestion tablets at the pharmacy".

Troy starts the truck up on his way to the school.

Chapter Six

"Metabolic disease" Ahmed ponders. "Is this why we're all getting fatter?". The robot continues churning out boxes that need labelling. Ahmed yawns and returns his attention to the hypertensive meds and sleeping pills or "Z drugs" the robot just spat out. He recognizes Troy's name.

Pharmacy is really changing Ahmed thinks. He casts his mind back. It's changing from moving boxes of pills. Lately he's seen the hype about weight loss injections (he knows them as GLP-1 receptor agonists) and he knows he's going to be asked about them. Again. Maybe he should look into that but perhaps there are other ways that don't mean more injections…

He doesn't mind doing injections or 'jabbing' as it's known in healthcare.

He was there at the front-line during the Covid-19 pandemic. Counting the injections in dozens each day. Looking back, it's hard to believe what it was like. People queuing out the door. No masks or gloves available. No one would believe you unless they'd been there at the time, he thought.

As he sticks the labels on Troy's boxes, he rubs his tired, scratchy eyes and wonders "Will we consider metabolic disease a threat like Covid-19?"
He'd read somewhere that managing chronic diseases like obesity, diabetes, and cardiovascular disease, could bankrupt economies.

The Uber takes Sarah home. She looks away, to avoid eye contact, as Troy's truck passes, on his way into the pharmacy parking lot.

The door swings open and into the pharmacy stumbles Troy. Good timing Ahmed thinks.

"Hi Troy", he calls. Ada is busy with another customer, discussing a blood pressure check, "How can I help?"

"Indigestion relief please", says Troy rubbing his chest. "It's bad".

Ahmed looks carefully at Troy and queries his symptoms. Getting Troy some generic indigestion relief, Ahmed urges Troy to consult his family physician.

Troy ambles back to his truck, slurping a mouthful of chalky, gooey stuff, "At least it tastes OK". Happily, the pain in his chest has eased a little.

For now.

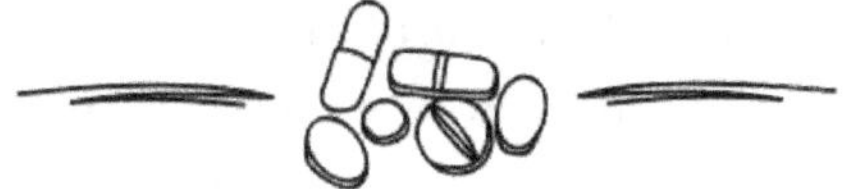

"I want my Mommy".

This is wrong and I don't like it.

"Where's Mommy? Where's Daddy?"

"Why are you telling me to go with these strangers?"

My name is Connie. I'm five.

"I WANT MY MOMMY!"

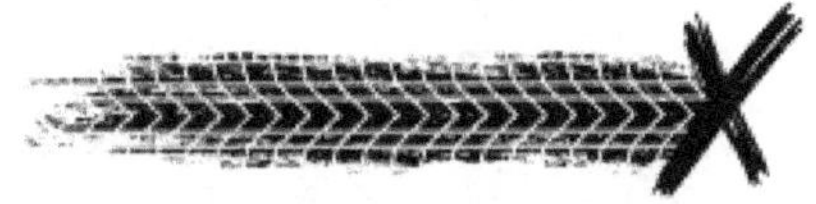

At school, it couldn't go much worse for the duo from social services. In the morning, after a call from the police, they had a long phone call with the headteacher. ID'd themselves on arrival and it seemed to be going about as well as could be expected.

Things go from bad to worse when the sister-in-law marches in and starts threatening to call the police. A shouting match ensues and at its crescendo, another teacher oblivious to the abysmal timing, brings Connie and Isla into the office.

Shouting, two little girls crying, Connie and Isla in the aunt's arms. It isn't supposed to be like this. While never 'fun' this is whole other level of wrong.

When some guy turns up delivering stationery, the Lead from social services rapidly decides to compromise, in an attempt to limit the damage. "And they wonder why I drink", she Mombles to herself as she rifles through her paperwork, looking for this form and that form.

Double-checking she has everyone's address, and everyone has signed. The two girls go home with the aunt.

Temporarily. Everyone crying.

Chapter Seven

"Ping, ping, ping", a series of text messages come through to the aunt's phone when she gets outside. It's Robert asking after the girls; bluntly stating Val is dead; demanding she calls back.

Connie and Isla climb into the car (her own kids are at home with her husband - so there are child seats).

Thinking fast, auntie says they'll go to McDonald's. She tries calling Robert, but it just goes to voicemail.

Sending a quick message "I've got the girls", she puts some music on and babbles away trying to distract them.

"Who's going to tell them their Mommy is dead?"

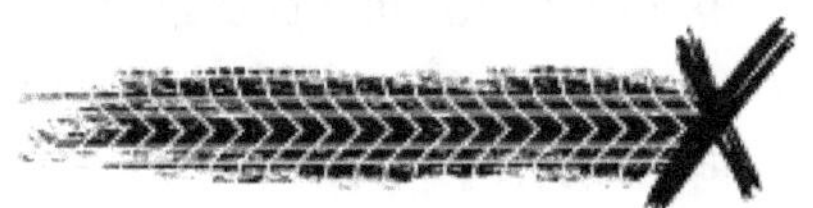

"Oh, me back", the pain trivializing the discomfort of the nylon wrap cutting into his hands, Troy half drops the boxes of printing paper at the last customer. The usual words exchanged, and delivery note passed over. Soon he's on his way back to the industrial park, fighting the late afternoon traffic.

"Maybe I should see the Doc about me heart. Ahmed said I should". His thoughts then turn to Robert after seeing the furor at the school, with both little girls and the teachers crying.

He'd made himself scarce.

Sometimes it's better to just get out of the way.

"I wonder what happened? And where's Sarah been all day?"

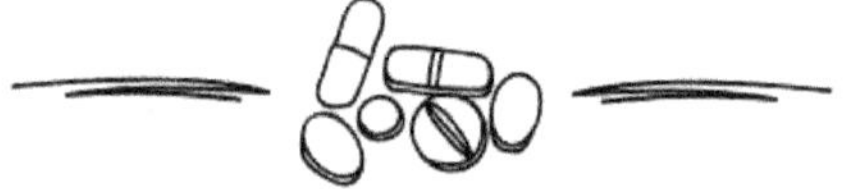

Robert returns to consciousness with competing thoughts. It's exhausting. His little girls and then Val. For a moment he tries to put Val out of his mind, but grief comes charging back and floors him.

The police say social services are looking after the girls. "My God, they're not going to understand that. Gotta get up".

Really, not wanting to eat, noticing the drip in his arm as if for the first time, he presses the button to call the nurse.

"Gotta get outta here. Now!" he declares to the nurse. "Get this bloody thing out me arm".

"OK be calm please, I'll page the physician, and we'll see if we can get you discharged. Please be still..." they whine on.

Robert's pulse racing, "What the f**k is going on?" His phone has no signal. Of course.

It began as just an ordinary day, he thought. Now Val's dead; the kids are with social services; and I'm in hospital.

"I wonder if Val's sister can help?".

Shock, disbelief and fear for his little girls, all vie for his attention. His blood sugar level is all over the place, the untouched meal on the tray beside him, slowly congeals.

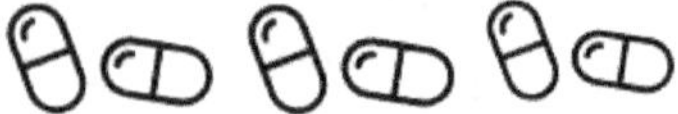

"Didn't know sleep was such a big deal..." Ahmed says laughing with the two guys on the stand at the Pharmacy Convention, bizarrely dressed in pajamas!

He struggled with insomnia himself some nights but hadn't put it all together.

When he slept badly, he knew he:

- Ate too much of the wrong things
- Felt tired and lazy
- Was grumpy and his whole body ached

Was that such a big deal?

The sheer scale of the sleep problem (in the multiple millions undiagnosed in his country alone) still missed him, and he didn't appreciate the interplay of sleep disorders and chronic diseases.

But something was nagging at the corner of his mind, as he left the convention. Not fully formed, he couldn't quite grasp it. Something joined this all up:

- Sarah's weight problem
- Troy's heart attack
- Robert's diabetes

But what could HE do about it? Was it even up to him? His subconscious played with it as he drove home.

Ahmed gets home late. His mind buzzing. He starts worrying about being tired tomorrow if he doesn't get enough sleep. So, predictably he tosses, turns, and struggles to get off to sleep. After waking multiple times, at 04:30hrs he gives up, puts the light on, and checks his phone.

But something has clicked into place. He can see the connections now.

Each of the three patients is a medical silo and each he suspects has an undiagnosed sleep disorder!

And he realizes that these patients all come to HIM. They are all there right in front of HIM. And there are millions more undiagnosed, just like them.

HE IS AWAKE NOW.

Chapter Eight

Thud.

The coroner closed his book.

Then looked through the glass at the body lying on the slab in the mortuary.

No. Not just 'A' body.

MY BODY.

I'm dead.

My name had been Helen. But you wouldn't have stopped and talked to me. I looked exactly what I was. A drug addict.

But I didn't want to die though. No, that was not part of my plan.

The coroner knew he had to rule my death 'accidental'. My death was just another in a rising and apparently unnoticed trend.

A trend called 'Pharming'. Sounded innocent enough if you were overheard. But it had nothing to do with tractors nor cows.

It meant 'hitting' one pharmacy after another until you had all you needed. Staying high for longer and dealing with the down was my purpose.

And 'sleep aids' were easy to get and dirt cheap. You just gave the pharmacy staff the same old lines and got a bit shirty if necessary. In the end, they always gave them to you, so you left and didn't cause a scene.

Then hit the next pharmacy. And the next one. No name needed. Nothing at all. Easy as shootin' heroin.

As long as you could pay.

You had to be careful though to get the right ones. They had long and complicated names. Diphenhydramine, Promethazine.

Don't screw up and get the non-drowsy ones. Waste of money. Yeah, OK so I was just another junkie.

And you don't give a damn.

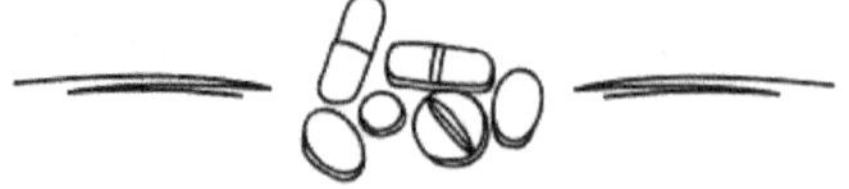

The coroner was seeing more and more cases like Helen's. Another drug overdose. 'Accidental'. But it grated.

Unless the police found something new, it was considered 'accidental' because Helen hadn't left a suicide note.

Helen had been combining opioid street drugs with sedating antihistamines or 'sleep aids', bought from several pharmacies.

But Helen had never struggled with insomnia.

Chapter Nine

"In a car while stopped for a few minutes in traffic?" asked Ahmed. "As with the other questions, if you haven't been in a car recently, try to determine how it would affect you".[2]

Zero went into the answer box.

Ahmed wasn't fooled.

They'd scored straight 3s for every other question. And he could see sitting here discussing sleepiness was a battle for them. Sleep was threatening to overtake them at any moment.

'Intelligent interpretation' was the phrase he'd heard on the sleep course.

Now he knew exactly what they'd meant. Vocational drivers and others, where their livelihood depended on them being alert, were hardly likely to say they were sleepy on the job!

---

[2] Ahmed is using the Epworth Sleepiness Scale. Johns MW. A new method for measuring daytime sleepiness: the Epworth Sleepiness Scale. Sleep. 1991;14(6):540-545

He'd heard their reasons before; getting help took 'forever' and who would want to wear that 'diving mask' thing in bed?!

So, Ahmed made a side note of his concerns as he continued through the Clinical Decision Support System questions, screening the patient for sleep apnea.

Outside the consulting room, he heard raised voices. Never a good sign he thought. He was momentarily torn between staying put, being professional and dealing with the person in front of him or intervening between Ada and 'shouty'.

When the swearing started, his decision was made for him.

Excusing himself, locking the screen of the computer, he hurriedly left the consulting room, but as he arrived the external door swung shut and a peculiar quiet descended.

Ada looked at him half reproachful, "where were you?" and half seeking forgiveness.

"What was that all about?" Asked Ahmed.
"Sleep aid request. And they didn't like me asking questions. Happens all the time. I should have known

better..." Ada's voice trailed off. Ahmed passes the tissues and suggests Ada take five and put the kettle on.

For a moment, the sound of snoring emanating from the consulting room brought his attention back to his "I'm not sleepy" consultation.

A glance at Ada wiping her eyes, as she passes him a cup of coffee, jerks him back to 'sleep aids'.

These 'sleep aids' are a damn menace he thought. Psychologically addictive and typically used for far longer than 'short-term'. And those that chose to, abused them, and pharmacy staff trying to help them.

Recognizing it for what it was: an ethical dilemma. Ahmed mused that he made money from selling 'sleep aids'. Not a lot perhaps, but it all helped when he was skimming along the bottom of his overdraft. He'd even noticed cough medicine had diphenhydramine in it.

Seems it's everywhere! Damn. Feeling conflicted he recalled the documentaries about the 'OxyRelief crisis' and couldn't fail to see the parallel.

But what to do?

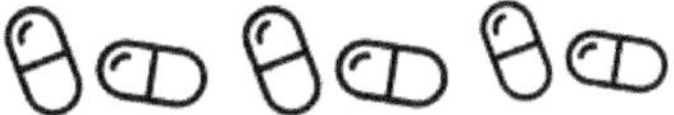

The Court summons lay on the kitchen table amidst the crumbs.

"This happens to other people", thought Sarah, "not me".

Sarah is going to trial. If she loses, against the charge of 'vehicular homicide', she faces a prison sentence.

She feels like she's watching herself in a movie. It just seems to get worse and worse. And she must pay for a lawyer now.

Disbelief left long ago, leaving her alone with misery and apathy. More comfort eating.

Sarah had been prescribed Positive Airway Pressure therapy for sleep apnea. The lawyer said that as her condition was undiagnosed at the time of the 'incident' (the police refused to say 'accident') it was a mitigating factor.

She wasn't holding her breath.

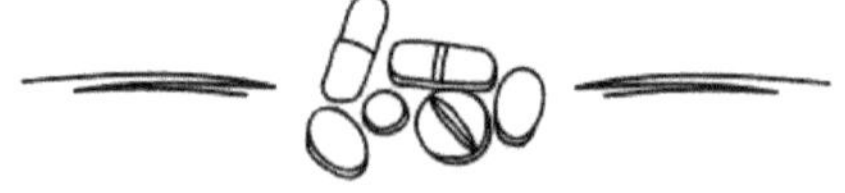

"Going anywhere nice this summer?" said the dentist with both hands in Ben's mouth, as they assessed the remains of an occlusion.

12 months ago, Ben, a recent graduate lawyer had kept his girlfriend, and now wife happy, by using an anti-snoring gadget. He'd used it every night.

And it had sort of worked.

For the snoring, "she married me after all".

But the consequences a year later had brought him to the dental chair. He could no longer bite with his front teeth.

And his jaw hurt like hell.

Ahmed the pharmacist had screened him for sleep apnea, advised him to have a home sleep apnea test, and said he should see his physician. After considering the cost of the sleep test, his student loan and going out Friday night, he decided "It's only snoring".

Ignoring Ahmed's advice, he bought a 'boil and bite' anti-snoring gadget. Ahmed sold them, so they had to be alright, he reasoned.

Ben's uncontrolled tooth movement was a thing of wonder. The dentist 'wondered' where to begin...

"Ok, so…", they sucked through their teeth like a second-hand car salesman being asked for a discount, "this is quite a mess I'm afraid".

"You now have an anterior open bite and unilateral temporomandibular joint dysfunction. We're into remedial work. And we'll need to replace this cracked bridge", they said tapping the 3-unit gold and porcelain restoration with the probe.

That one had cost Ben more than he cared to remember. Ben visualized the money floating through the air from his wallet across the room to the dentist's.

Shortly afterwards, in the dental reception area, gulping as he contemplated the invoice and the proposed year of 'remedial' dental work. He raced through malpractice and consumer protection law in his head and considered if Ahmed was liable.

Looking up, Ben noticed a leaflet for a custom-made, anti-snoring device. Remarking to the dentist, reviewing the next patient's notes, "Wouldn't recommend one of them then!"

The dentist rolled his eyes… not prepared to take the time to explain the difference.

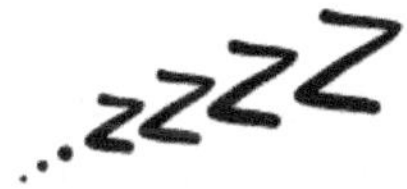

The next morning, as Sarah awoke feeling rested and took off her PAP therapy mask, she had an idea. She smiled to herself for the first time in ages.

"Hello Ahmed", said Robert as he wiped his feet on the entrance mat.

"Hi Robert. How are you?" Ahmed replies, noting the pressure lines across Robert's cheeks.

"Inside me nose is real sore. Want some Vaseline".

"Oh no Robert. Don't use that. That could cause pneumonia! Let's have a look at you. Would you come this way please?" Ahmed beckons Robert to the consulting room.

Ahmed asks, "So, how's it going with Positive Airway Pressure therapy? Sleeping better? Feeling any more rested?"

"I've had loads of scary dreams" says Robert. "A bit off-putting to be honest. And my nose is killing me. It's sore inside. Here..." he says, spreading his nose across his face, so Ahmed can see his red and sore nasal septum.

Ahmed, explaining about REM sleep rebound, glances up Robert's nose.

"Yes, I see", he says, making some notes. "I've noticed a couple of other things. Robert, you're over-tightening the mask straps. It's a classic error. And we need to get you some humidification. That will sort your nose".

Ahmed elaborates about keeping his mask clean and letting the air cushion inflate.

On his way out the door, Robert brushes past Troy coming in. They don't know each other.

They're both luckier than they know. They owe a great deal to Ahmed. They're diagnosed and getting treatment.

Because of him.

Unlike 80% of people with undiagnosed sleep apnea, who go unrecognized and untreated.

,zZZz   ,zZZz   ,zZZz

Sarah hires the community center. The date is set. Ada (who's in on Sarah's secret plan), invites Ahmed to join her and Troy at home for a dinner party just to reserve the date. She puts it on the work calendar and won't let Ahmed forget.

Surreptitiously working with Ada and the physicians from the surrounding area, Sarah hopes everyone Ahmed has helped with their sleep over the years, learns of their plan.

But not Ahmed!

Noting that each patient typically has a partner whose sleep has improved as well, Sarah has no real clue how many people to expect.

Chapter Ten

"Can I have a word please?"

Ben says quietly in the pharmacy. Ada after a few preliminary questions, asks him to take a seat.

Expecting to wait, Ben has barely sat down, when Ahmed invites him to the consulting room.

Ben explains his jaw pain and dental issues, and how the dentist said it was caused by the 'boil and bite' anti-snoring gadget, he'd purchased from Ahmed.

"Outside the bounds of his scope of practice".

Not a happy day.

Later, Ahmed withdraws the anti-snoring devices from sale.

He had never heard of the MAUDE database before today.

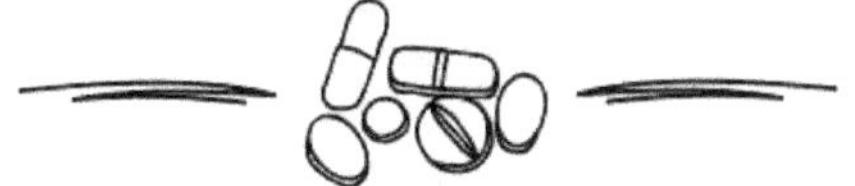

He can't recall where he learned about it, perhaps a physician mentioned it... But Ahmed discovers that a smartphone app providing 'Cognitive Behavioral Therapy for Insomnia' known as CBT-I, is now the first approach recommended for insomnia.

The irony of delivering help for insomnia on a mobile phone didn't miss Ahmed.

He's learned it's more than the often touted 'sleep hygiene' concept and 'they made it free so everyone can access it'.

"How does making it free mean everyone can access it then?" He sighs.

Ahmed pondered the realities of his fledgling sleep service, the insomnia sufferers that keep coming, and his dwindling reserves.

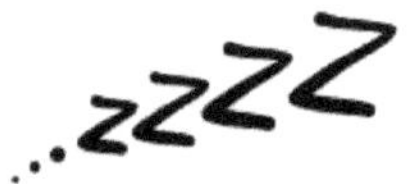

The cub reporter for the local news yawned, stretched and noticed the stain on his trousers from lunch.

"Hell…", he was bored.

Maybe this afternoon something newsworthy would happen? Shop lifting had filled his morning, and his editor would wonder what he'd been doing all day. As the case for the prosecution was read out, he forgot his numb backside and started his covert voice recording.

Scribbling frantically, he thought "finally!"

"… the decedent…," said the lawyer, enunciating each syllable with precision. And continued detailing the question of whether the driver had caused death because they had fallen asleep.

Sarah, nervously swallowed, as she was sworn in with one hand on the bible. Her head pounding, she felt weak, sick and was having trouble speaking. The eyes of a man in the public gallery bore into her.

Robert was doing all he could not to either start crying or shouting as he stared at the woman, who allegedly had killed his wife, and robbed his daughters of their mother.

Glancing about him, the reporter could feel the electricity in the air. His pen moved rapidly across the page; the words flowing. He couldn't stop to wonder if his editor would run the story. He just had to present something. Something to show his editor and thank them for the faith they'd shown, giving him a job in the first place.

Sarah collapses.

For a moment nobody moves. Then suddenly, everyone is running around and shouting over each other.

At first, they think she fainted.

But when the medics arrive and Sarah is unresponsive, they suspect either a stroke or brain hemorrhage.

Sarah, although recently diagnosed with sleep apnea, had struggled using positive airway pressure therapy.

In the ambulance, despite desperate efforts by the paramedics, Sarah is pronounced dead.

The reporter has his story.

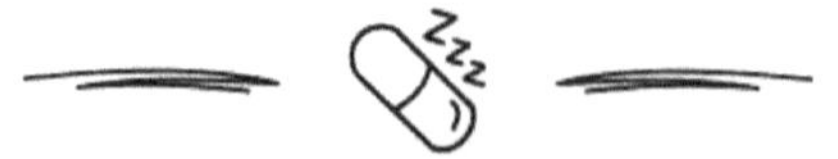

"Oh my God I feel so much better! Amazing, sleep can do that for you!" Troy enthuses.

"You know I thought it was a right load of... psychobabble. But you get out of it what you put in. Thanks, Ahmed, for encouraging me to stick with it. Gotta say, I wouldn't have persisted without you".

Troy had used the CBT-I app Ahmed recommended, alongside his PAP-machine for sleep apnea and now he wanted help getting off the 'Z' drugs.

Ahmed said he'd become 'habituated' to them.

While Ahmed was delighted the app had helped; the naïve 'free' pricing strategy left no room to compensate his pharmacy for supporting insomnia sufferers like Troy. "Dumb", he Mumbled, "this is where people are".

Of course, Ahmed would help Troy. Despite it being another 'invisible' service, he didn't get paid for, that saved everyone money. He was just wired that way. He cared.

Ahmed's professional reputation was growing. Happy people talked about him. Wives sent their husbands. Physicians referred their patients.

Robert and Troy were still alive because of him.

Preferring to take the minor financial 'hit' and not have Ada abused by addicts, he no longer stocked 'sleep aids'. Or certain brands of cough medicine, for that matter.

Legitimate insomnia issue or direct product requests were directed to him. He knew menopausal women declaring insomnia symptoms could well have sleep apnea.

"Men and women are different", he smiled to himself.

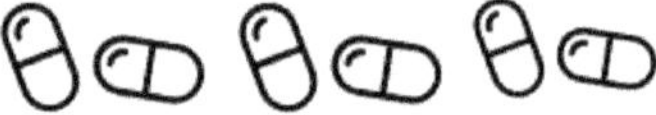

The irony made Ahmed give a wry smile. All these initiatives and entrepreneurial support schemes. And he seemed to qualify for none of them. He was just doing it.

Becoming cynical for a moment he thought "I can't be alone in wondering why we don't appreciate sleep? When inadequate sleep is the thread that connects chronic diseases…"

Ahmed's success with his sleep service had become first regional and then national news. While the businessman in him valued the publicity, he wasn't comfortable in front of a camera or microphone.

So, when the cub reporter came asking questions about Sarah, they got absolutely nowhere. As if he was going to discuss patient confidential matters with a journalist!

But it made him wonder… it was an awful situation.

"I need you to leave", he says.

"But did you know Sarah's dead?" the cub reporter replied.

Ahmed's face told the reporter all he needed to know.

Chapter Eleven

Time passes. And the day dawns a beautiful golden yellow, as Ahmed's rising profile for helping sleep patients, leads him to receive an invitation to take part in a clinical trial of an innovative, oral drug to treat sleep apnea.

Yes! In his community pharmacy. He's proud and confident he's helping people.

The drug company explain that a geographic spread of pharmacies across the country should make the results more reliable.

"Sounds amazing! Imagine not having to struggle with PAP or anti-snoring devices". One pill a day and no more sleep apnea.

"That would be a winner," he remarked. "Everyone would want that."

Ahmed enthusiastically enrolls and commits his pharmacy's time and resources.

The trial runs for a few months and despite the disruption to his normal pharmacy routine, Ahmed feels it's worthwhile.

Ahmed isn't stupid. 'Therapeutic failure' is how he'd term it.

The results he records are not positive. Basically, the drug doesn't work.

Sad.

But he's a stickler, "it's really important to accurately record the data."

Wondering if perhaps his patient group are the placebo control arm, (meaning his patients had no active ingredients in their pills) he moves on to other things.

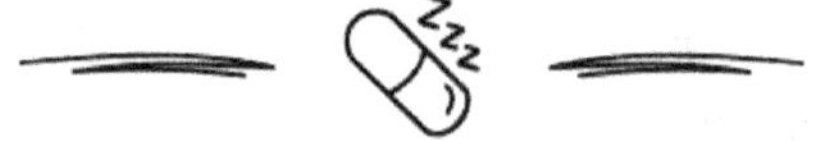

Robert feels like a new man. Ten years younger. He's doing some exercise, lost weight (thanks Ahmed) and has a new wife. An expanded family. His diabetes is well controlled now he's on PAP and each year the PAP mask technology improves and gets easier to tolerate.

Val crosses his mind from time to time. He's only human. Every evening his girls mention Mommy as he tucks them into bed, and his new wife doesn't know where to put herself.

Maybe one day it won't cut so much.

$$_z z^Z z \quad _z z^Z z \quad _z z^Z z$$

The postponed party for Ahmed finally happens. Though a bitter-sweet affair with both Sarah and Val dead, he is the man of the moment.

"Hold her hair back Connie!" As cake, fizzy drink, and half-digested sweets reappear. Isla vomits profusely.

The party is overwhelming for Ahmed. On the one hand, he can't voice his happiness. What a lovely thing to do!

On the other, should he risk everything going up against the pharmaceutical company proclaiming a successful pill to treat sleep apnea?

Their published results certainly don't reflect his experience of their drug.

Every night his mind plays it over and over. Haunting him in the witching hours.

Robert, Val, the girls, Sarah.

Could he have been there for Sarah?

He'd found his purpose — he was on a mission to transform lives through better sleep.

Chapter Twelve

"CLOSED".

Does that mean closed for lunch? But it's not ten in the morning?! Troy stared blankly at the red sign on the door, unable to fully comprehend its message.

Now what?

He'd tried phoning the family physician's clinic and hung up when he got an automated service. Press 1 for "Goodbye" and 2 to "Get lost" he thought.

What was he supposed to do now? There were no others to go to. And directing him to a telephone service just wound him up. It was like pulling teeth.

Why didn't they have access to his records and stop asking daft questions?

"I will go see Ahmed".

They said his services were 'Patient centric' in the articles written about him.

Ahmed set up his sleep service a few years ago now. Over time it had mutated into a metabolic health center. He did it to help people and felt he had merely recognized what was staring him in the face.

"All this 'talk' of moving hospital services to primary care", he thought.

Not a bitter man, Ahmed, browsed through the letters and leaflets in the mail. Social prescribing was the latest 'in thing', shame it's not joined up "Can't believe they don't understand, I'm not funded to provide a patient facing service".

There are only so many hours in the day he mused. And now the family physician's clinic has closed.

Time.

It all comes back to time, sighed Ahmed.

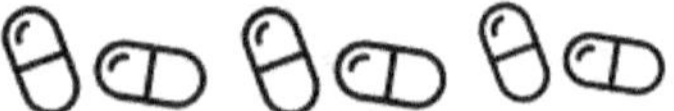

The second au pair (the first having left after three weeks) herds the children to the car.

"Put seatbelts on plezzz" she commands in a European accent, while loading their multiple bags and water bottles into the car.

Another school day begins for Isla and Connie.

"They're remarkable", thinks Robert. "They've just got on with it". Less and less, the death of 'Mommy' comes up in conversation.

Robert must be there at bedtime.

That is non-negotiable.

Cuddles, bedtime stories and prescription melatonin.

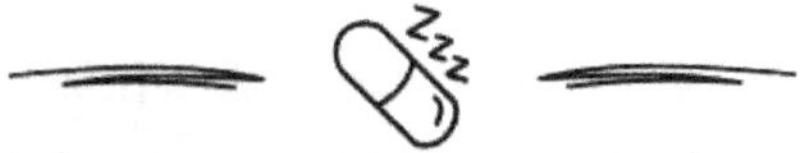

Ahmed is jerked back to the moment as a furious Troy bangs open the pharmacy door.

"Hello Troy", says a cautious Ada. "How can I help?"

Sensing an issue, Ahmed strolls round the low wall and takes over the conversation. Ada resumes where she left off.

"They've closed the bloody clinic!"

"I heard".

"What we supposed to do?"

"Well, there are telephone and online…" … "That don't help", interrupts Troy. "Need to speak to someone who knows me medical 'istory and can touch where it bloody hurts. They can't do that over the bloody phone!"

"OK Troy, come with me. I'm here to help you", Ahmed says calmly, guiding the irate Troy to the consulting room.

Once again, in a very similar way to when pharmacy was there during the CV-19 pandemic, pharmacy selflessly steps up as a sector.

To help people. And they have the gall to describe pharmacists as 'failed physicians'.

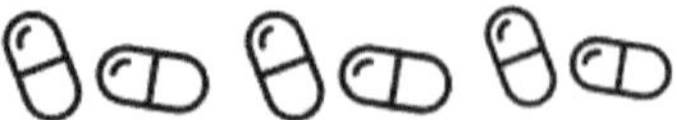

That night, sleep comes and goes.

Ahmed is awake.

Again.

But something is different. It's more than his usual mourning Val and Sarah.

He can't put his finger on it at first, and then he realizes the clock has frozen.

He'd been watching the numbers relentlessly progress:

03:35hrs.

"It's all about time", he thought.

Time to do this, time to do that.

Time to take your pills.

Time to wake up.

Time to go.

Part Two

My name is SLEEP, a part of you,
A piece of every creature true.
Yet I'm abused, taken for granted,
My value often disenchanted.

But every now and then, I rise,
With spectacles that stun your eyes.
Or subtle hints, a gentle prod,
I'm almighty like a God.

If you ignore or disrespect,
My power you shall not neglect.
For I will strike, a force unkind,
And leave my mark upon your mind.

So, heed this warning, don't forget,
Abuse me not, or you'll regret.
For SLEEP is vital, pure and deep,
Respect me, and your health you'll keep.

Sarah collapsed.

There was only the sound of her limbs hitting the woodwork on the way down. Then a deafening silence. For a pregnant moment everything stopped and then just as suddenly, reality rushed back in with a vengeance. Everyone shouting.

The reporter, forgetting himself, had mentally joined the scene and then remembered he was meant to be witnessing the event.

His pen restarted. He reminded himself that he was a professional. Young maybe, but Sarah's story had caught his editor's attention, and he'd been noticed because of it.

Sam was going to follow this story even more closely now.

His story hadn't died.

It had just begun.

"Let's see what you're made of". Said SLEEP.

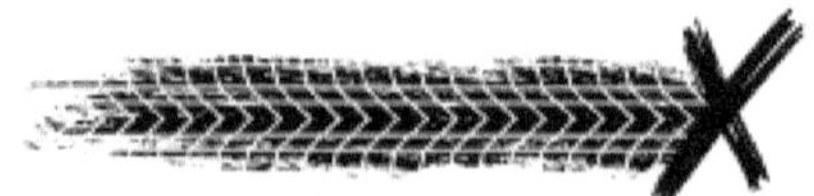

To look at her lying there, she appeared fine. Unconscious, clothes and hair in disarray but otherwise OK.

What the experienced eyes of the paramedics' saw was somewhat different.

Sarah had not fainted.

Unresponsive. Pupils fixed and dilated, clammy skin, and vital signs that all added up to 'scoop and run'.

"She didn't respect me." Spat SLEEP.

₂zZz   ₂zZz   ₂zZz

'Beep, beep, beep'.

The dead man's switch woke him. Almost immediately he could feel himself going again, fight against it as he did, his eyes closed.

03:35hrs, he was fast asleep despite the noise and vibration of the train he was driving.

It happened every morning. At pretty much the same point. Jerking awake once more, he took another slug of 'energy drink' and fully opened the side window, to get a blast of cold air into his face.

"They say we run these freight trains at night", he thought "because the railway lines are less busy with commuters". Certainly, IronLine Freight trains are long and slow. However, he'd heard their noise, and vibration affected the sleep of everyone along their route.

And he had to stay awake to drive it.

Least that was the idea.

"I'm going to bite him." Said SLEEP.

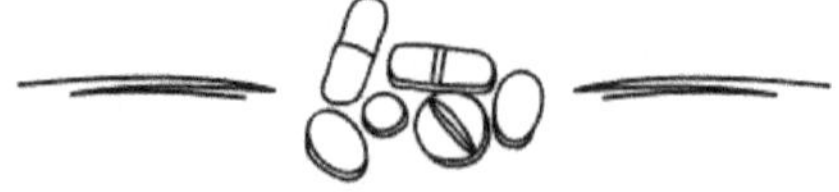

She fiddled with the pen.

Click, click. *Pause*. Click, click. *Pause*.

Faith had a problem. Actually, her employer had a problem. And she was effectively IronLine Freight's moral compass. The trouble was her message conflicted with the management's short-sighted, annual financial plan.

It was called 'short-termism'. She'd just call it dumb. Why couldn't they see? It was an accident waiting to happen. An annual target meant her argument for longer-term thinking was 'unwelcome'.

Click, click. *Pause*. Click, click. *Pause*.

Like a heartbeat.

"She shows promise. I will follow this one with interest". Mused SLEEP.

Toni read the news article. She'd loosely followed Ahmed's story about his sleep screening service in the pharmacy trade press. It had planted a seed at the back of her mind.

Anyone could see that a tragic story like Sarah's would inspire Ahmed. But Toni wasn't sure if she could replicate it in her pharmacy. It was new and unproven, and it differed from moving boxes.

- Demand?
- Costs?

Too many unknowns.

Closing the news app, she read about GLP-1 receptor agonists, or 'get thin' injections, in the trade news app. Failing to see the connection with sleep.

"Maybe. Just maybe". Pondered SLEEP.

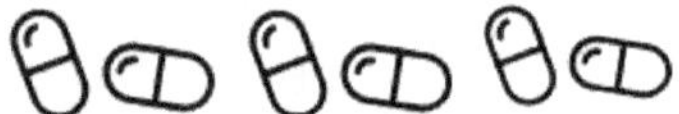

Sam looked beneath the lid.

Was even so bold as to lift the lid on the problem.

Sleep apnea was not recorded as the cause of death. Sarah's death was recorded as a brain hemorrhage.

"Something odd there", he thought. His curious mind sensing something.

The reporter had done his homework, and he knew Sarah's sleep apnea condition affected millions of people, yet 80% were undiagnosed.

"Why then was Sarah's cause of death not recorded as untreated sleep apnea?"

Sam would find out.

"Ooh. He's daring. I like him". Thought SLEEP.

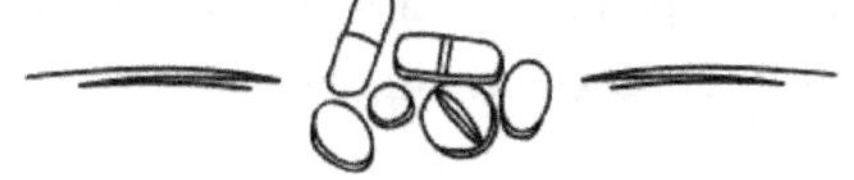

It's the annual Pharmacy Convention.

The usual hubbub and stands with the usual stuff and the usual messages.

Except, Toni recalled last year there was a sleep charity here. With a tiny stand and some people in pajamas. She'd take a look. Maybe they could explain how Ahmed made it work and whether it was worth a go.

Or if she was lucky, she could meet Ahmed himself. She weaved her way through the crowded gangways between stands dodging the lurking reporter.

"She's on the right track". Delighted SLEEP.

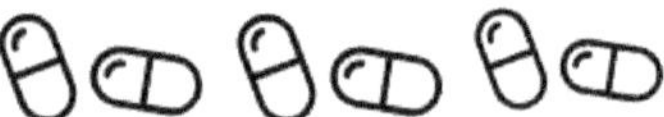

"So, the report shows that what they call the 'primary cause of death' was a brain hemorrhage, right?" murmured Sam. Deep in thought.

"Yup", said Faith.

"But that misses the point". He paused and then continued, "Sarah fell asleep and crashed. Val died at the scene and later Sarah died in the court room, all

because Sarah had untreated sleep apnea. To me it's the other way around".
"Well, you're not the coroner", snapped Faith, looking up from the coroner's report.

"You see, the coroner reports the 'direct mechanism' of death" she continued.

"I wonder how often that happens..." Sam almost audibly thought. Immune to her bad mood.

Eyes rolling, Faith knew Sam wouldn't let it go.

"It's a bit like Covid-19. Seems they don't record it as the cause..."

He's not listening to me and they're not listening at work.

"Story of my life", she Mombled.

"Keep going Sam." Thought SLEEP.

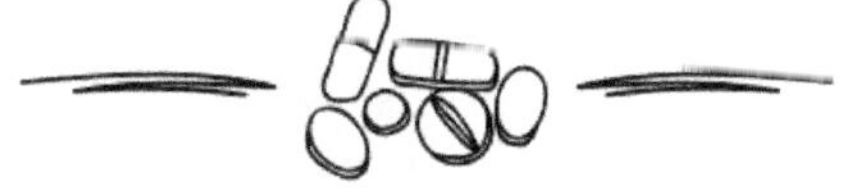

'Human Factors, Director, Faith Drew' it said on her office door.

The term 'Human Factors' always struck Faith as cold and dispassionate. As if people were merely a cog in a machine or from a viewpoint where tolerance for people's fallibility should be calculated like maxiMom sustainable revolutions or miles per gallon.

It was all about money.

Or how hard we can push people before they break. Sleep therefore was seen as an inconvenient cost burden.

"YES! You're starting to get it Faith. But what are you going to DO about it?" queried SLEEP.

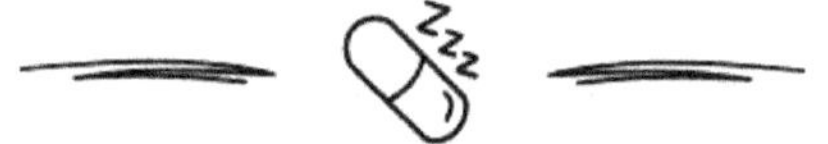

Faith and Sam had been seeing each other for about a year now. So, when Sam moved the conversation on to the impact of drowsiness upon safety at work, her eyebrows nearly disappeared off the top of her head.

That was one of 'those' questions. One she couldn't even mention at work. The 'elephant in the room'.

Sarah's death and the inquest findings had them both exploring the impact of sleep on productivity. In the evenings and on weekends. They could help each other. Their professional and personal interests now aligned. Sam was listening to her.

His job was to find the stories that mattered. He bought his ticket online for the pharmacy convention, hoping his Editor would approve reimbursement. He was going anyway.

That night or was it morning... the 03.35hrs train rumbled past as usual. Triggering insomnia for some. Faith and Sam though were lucky. Despite their sleep being fragmented, they turned over and went back to sleep. Then forgot all about it.

"BINGO! So, just to prove I'm not all bad, I played nicely, see?" posed SLEEP.

"Fine, I'll prove it then. I'll build a business case for sleep. Will you help me, Sam?"

"Sure. What's a business case?"

"Ok…" I say, trying hard not to sigh and roll my eyes "it's the money argument for doing something".

"Oh", he replies. None the wiser.

I guess I'm on my own here.

"Sam, this will help us. But there's a lot to do and the board meeting is…"

I pause and think. Damn it's in a month's time. That won't fly. Ok we'll aim for the next one.

"Sam, we've got 4 months. I will need your help".

"Tell me what to do".

So, I tell him we need to outline the financial impact. Yeah, I know there's more to a business case than that, but that's all the management want to read… if they get past the exec summary that is…

I dive in with my willing, if less than capable, helper... ChatGPT here I come. I'm going to need a pro account.

"This is fantastic! Keep going Faith."

"Hey Ahmed", I said in hope more than expectation, when I spot him at the sleep charity stand. Not that I've been loitering by the stand waiting for him. Honestly...

"Hello..." he says. Not recognizing me.

"I'm Sam, I work for the Bayside Herald. We met some time ago when... err..."

"Oh yes. I remember now", he saves me, but then a look of disgust crosses his face. "Look I've nothing to say. I told you..."

"No" I interrupt "I get that – absolutely respect that. I was a fool. Sorry. I was hoping to apologize and understand more about what you're doing".

"Oh".

I ploughed on and managed to win him round. Well maybe that's an exaggeration. Let's agree I got him to at least not hate me and accept my good intentions.

He thaws a little over a coffee and I explain that I'm planning to write a piece about his sleep screening service. What I neglected to say was that anything I learn will help Faith.

Maybe. At the very least his is a fascinating story, and as I've been swotting up on sleep disorders, I explain that I now get the scale of the issue. Hoping I don't get out of my depth as he clearly knows much more than me.

"I wonder..." pondered SLEEP.

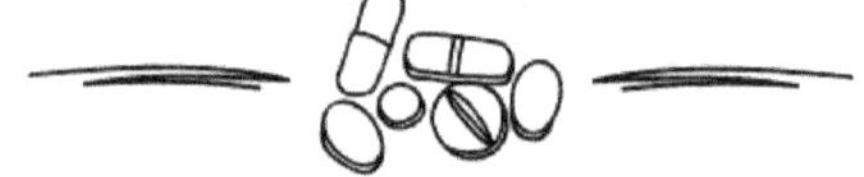

My boss likes the business case.

Wow!

But tells me not to get my hopes up.

He says it means change and whichever way you package it, change costs money. And in a competitive market yadda, yadda... you get the idea.

The board meeting comes around and I get to present it. I've made a PowerPoint. Got little sleep tinkering with it last night.

Yeah, I'm nervous.

"Told you!" Said SLEEP.

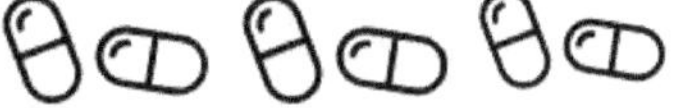

Faith's executive summary was a thing of beauty.

Shifting freight train operations from nighttime to daytime hours offered several benefits including: energy efficiency, enhanced safety, employee wellbeing, community consideration.

Blah, blah, blah.

"That is very good."
"They better listen…because I will be watching".

To my astonishment they listened. Bloody hell they even liked it! Asked some awkward questions and I was a little hazy on some answers. Said I'd find out. They seemed positive.

I need a shower I'm sweaty.

Got to answer their questions in a presentation at the next meeting.

Can't quite believe it. Little ol' me, Faith Drew. Getting respect for sleep onto IronLine Freight's agenda.

One nil for Human Factors.

The soddin' 03:35hrs train woke us both as usual. But this time insomnia bit me. Sam just turned over and went back to sleep - of course.

"Now I want to see them deliver on their fine words."
Growled SLEEP.

An excited and optimistic Faith presented her follow up answers to IronLine Freight's board. She'd developed the business case into a comprehensive 'sleep and productivity' report.

The board fudged making decisions. Kicked it down the street. She was gutted. Angry. Felt misled and a personal failure.

Three months go past, and the accountants kill it. Faith's card is marked at work. She dared to ask 'the' question. Sleep was obviously dispensable and if people didn't like the way the company operated, they were free to leave.

'Churn', as in staff turnover, was at 'acceptable levels.' Acceptable to whom precisely was unclear. It was business as usual.

Suck it up buttercup.

The 03:35hrs train saw Faith awake and staring at the clock. Worrying about how shattered she'd be in the day. She loved her job and Human Factor roles were not that common. A new job meant moving home. Insomnia was now her constant companion.

"SLEEP does not take prisoners".

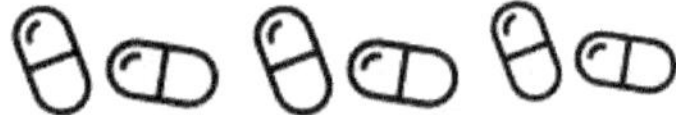

The long, hot summer continued and the roadworks outside Mike's house kept waking him up.

Earplugs helped but the heat inside with the windows closed rapidly became oppressive. Now as the noise from the roadworks entered the second week, he was tired going off to work at 9pm.

At the inquest after the train crash, they found no evidence of Mike having a sleep disorder.

In report speak he'd 'suffered a loss of awareness'. Which to everyone else meant he'd fallen asleep.

While IronLine Freight's marketing director began the process of rebranding to lose the negative impact on the company, the inquest found no evidence of wrongdoing.

However, an IronLine Freight, internal report was leaked to the press. Accompanying paperwork detailed how they'd dismissed on cost grounds, a pioneering approach from their own Human Factors department, to abolish night freight trains.

"Now it's getting interesting", smiled SLEEP.

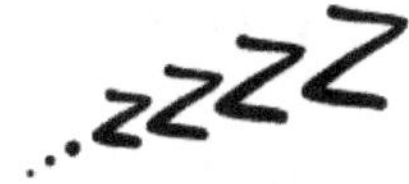

'Knock, knock'.

This time it was Jimmy's turn.

The police officer had the job of letting the family know.

It happened with a certain regularity. Perhaps every three to four months. A truck would crash on the highway that led from the industrial park where the courier and freight companies were based. Always in the wee hours.

Jimmy had fallen asleep while driving.

The paramedics knew. Didn't need a forensic examination. The obliteration of the front of the vehicle, perhaps against the leg of a bridge, the hour of the morning, no other vehicles nor skid marks on the road.

The location was excellent for business. Drivers could get on the highway network within minutes of leaving. Get to where things needed to be rapidly. But the lack of sleep, horrible hour of the morning and monotony of highway driving, periodically led to events like these.

Dog yapping, a smell of toast and coffee, the woman standing at the doorway in her nightie.

Kids calling, "Who is it Mom?"

The police officer swallowed hard and stuck to her script.

"Hate to say it... But I told you so".

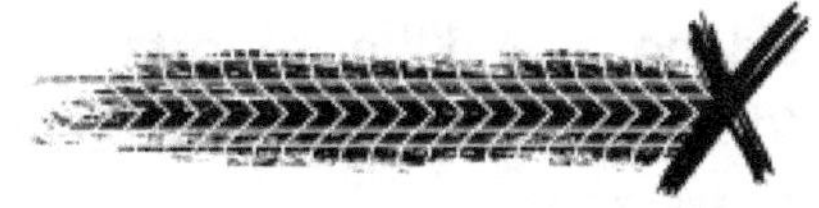

The day the news broke Faith and Sam had a massive row. In the usual way, copies of Faith's report had found their way to the investigative journalists of the national media.

"Look, if you'll just listen".

"No Sam", she interrupts "It's in my contract, I cannot talk to the media!"

"Hang on".

"Well, where the hell else did it come from Sam? I've already been summoned to HQ and my email and phone shut down".

She paused for breath in between shouts. "This is insane Sam. I will never get another job!"

Faith, met with IronLine management and was predictably put on gardening leave pending a full investigation.

IronLine Freight sent out the PR person while management hid and pointed fingers at each other. Sam left to stay with friends, hoping it would blow over. Yes, he'd 'borrowed' her report... and at the time thought she'd be angry at first, but then he'd explain, and she'd understand.

He felt lost without her.

"Patience. Wheels are turning". Thought SLEEP.

"You did WHAT?!"

"It's policy Ma'am. When someone is being dismissed, sorry put on gardening leave, we..." The HR department had taken Faith's phone and cut her off from the IT system within minutes of the exiting her decision being made.

"Well, how do we contact her now then?" The exasperated CEO asked.

"We write her a letter".

"Seriously? In this day and age? Fine".

Which of course meant anything but.

So, a letter was sent to Faith 'requesting' she meet with the CEO at a hotel near her home. No flexibility on date and time was offered.

In a remarkable feat of management gymnastics, worthy of any MBA graduate, IronLine Freight invited Faith to take on a new expanded Human Factors department. She'd have the corner office, and a pay rise etc. In return, IronLine Freight would get off the 'hook' of their own making.

Human Factors, Vice President, Faith Drew, it said on her office door.

She'd start by calling Sam.

"Well, there's a turnaround!" said a delighted SLEEP.

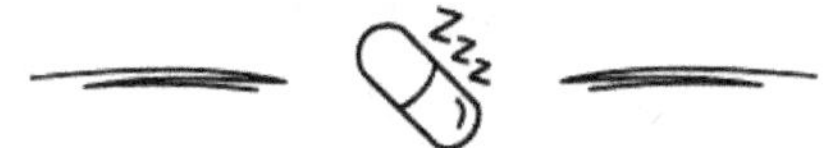

Ahmed and Sam met several times over the following months. Sam explained IronLine Freight's motivation to become an employer of choice, a company that appreciated the importance of sleep for productivity and safety. It helped Ahmed see that Sam was more than a newshound.

Ahmed's metabolic syndrome service had moved the traditional pharmacy business into the background.

Ada was still with him, and they had gradually expanded. Ahmed had big plans, money in the bank and time to think about his next step.

Sam's Editor grudgingly admired his story and without openly saying so, hinted he'd push it to the mainstream media and TV.

"This has legs", he said.

"Excellent Sam". Said SLEEP.

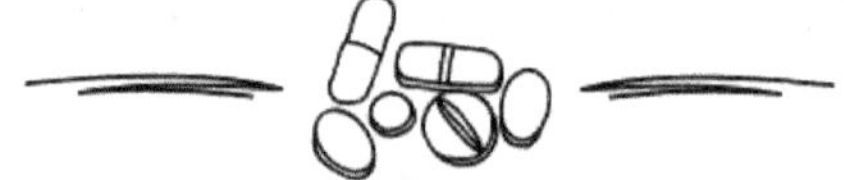

"That's fantastic Faith! I'm so pleased for you".

Sam was delighted with her news and relieved to hear from her again. Now was not the moment to talk about the leak of the report.

"They give VP to anyone now", said Sam, teasing her. He was so proud of her.

As she went to reply, he said "next they'll promote someone to VP of Paperclips".

"Sam...!" Faith exclaimed in mock outrage.

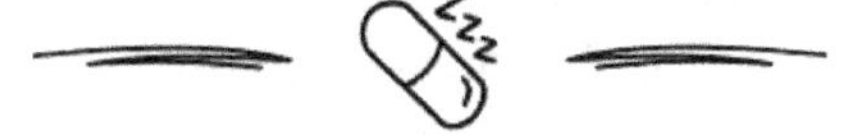

"Ahmed!" called the stand sponsor above the background noise of the convention.

"Oh hi", said Ahmed.

"I wanted to introduce you to Toni".

The usual chitchat ensued and Ahmed and Toni, without the businessman, wander off for a coffee.

Toni is full of questions. Ahmed likes to help. He runs through how he began small and how he slowly made it work. He relays how it all began with the terrible incident when Sarah fell asleep and killed Val.

They agree to talk again after the convention. And just before they part, Toni drops the bomb into the conversation.

She's Val's sister.

"Word is spreading of my value". Said SLEEP.

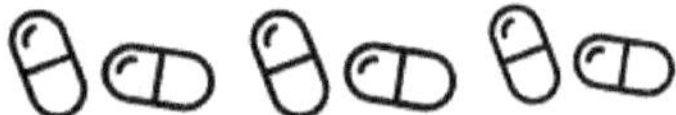

Jimmy or 'Bubba' as his friends knew him, was at his happiest in his truck. He loved his wife and kids. Even their daft dog when he was home. But driving was his day-to-day existence, and it made him feel alive and free.

He played by the rules. Mostly. And when he didn't, he made sure he didn't get caught. Nobody got hurt and he felt righteous in circumventing 'idiocy'.

The company's proposed 'in cab monitoring' threatened to invade his space and felt like a violation. GPS tracking, he said at the time they installed it, was the thin end of the wedge.

Admitting to feeling drowsy at work was to Jimmy a sign of weakness. "Can't stand the heat – get out of the kitchen". Jimmy was a solid, dependable trucker.

Sleep was for the weak.

Until he fell asleep, crashed and died. Widowing his wife. And leaving his kids without their 'Bubba'.

"Do you need another reminder?"

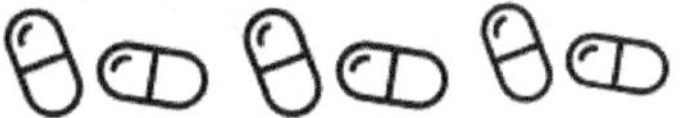

The End.

If you've been affected by anything in this book, whether it's bullying, asthma, depression, insomnia, sleep apnea, snoring, ADHD, or PTSD-related sleep disturbances, know that you're not alone and help is available.

Remember, you deserve restful sleep. Ask for help and take steps towards improving your sleep and well-being.

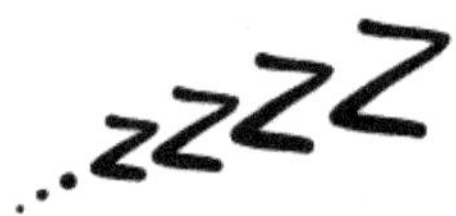

If you're a healthcare professional interested in helping people with perhaps undiagnosed sleep issues, then please do seek independent and evidence-based sleep education.

The BSPSS (British Society of Pharmacy Sleep Services) is a charitable incorporated organization providing free online sleep education for pharmacy professionals: https://bspss.org

The pharmacist character Ahmed uses the Snorer Pharmacy® Clinical Decision Support System to screen sleep issue individuals: https://snorer.com/pharmacist/

About the author

Adrian Zacher MBA is a distinguished expert in the sleep industry with over 30 years' experience.

As CEO and founder of the British Society of Pharmacy Sleep Services (BSPSS) a registered charitable incorporated organization, he is dedicated to making sleep expertise accessible through community pharmacies.

A portion of the proceeds from each book sale will be donated to support BSPSS initiatives, including:

- Providing sleep education and support to community pharmacists and their patients

- Raising awareness about the importance of healthy sleep and the risks associated with untreated sleep disorders

- Advancing research and best practices in the field of sleep medicine.

Also, by Adrian Zacher:

Killer in your Bedroom.
A concise, no-nonsense guide that empowers snorers and their partners to find evidence-based solutions for snoring and sleep apnea, while exposing ineffective gadgets and bureaucratic obstacles.

https://amzn.eu/d/bVF9cFE

Five inexpensive sleep information 'how to' guides available on Amazon.

https://www.amazon.co.uk/dp/B09NDTSTH1?binding=kindle_edition&ref_=ast_author_bsi

A textbook chapter in Carranza's Clinical Periodontology about sleep and the role of the dentist.

Reference information

Manufacturer and User Facility Device Experience (MAUDE) Database:
https://www.accessdata.fda.gov/scripts/cdrh/cfdocs/cfmaude/search.cfm

'Gumshields' for snoring
https://www.atsjournals.org/doi/full/10.1164/rccm.2007 01-114OC#.V9ukcFT_rio

'Sleep Aids'
Diphenhydramine and promethazine are among many first-generation sedating antihistamines developed to treat allergies, hay fever, and cold symptoms. They work by blocking the effects of histamine, a chemical released by the body during an allergic reaction.

Due to the side effect of sedating properties, these antihistamines are commonly used off-label as OTC (Over the Counter) 'sleep aids'.

Precautions and Limitations
While commonly used off-label, they have significant limitations and should only be used occasionally under the guidance of a healthcare provider.

Behavioral changes (CBT-I as relayed in the story) and approved insomnia medications are safer and more appropriate options for persistent sleep problems.

Precautions and limitations include:

- Tolerance to the sedative effects may develop quickly with repeated use.

- They may cause grogginess, dizziness, and impaired cognitive function the next day.

- Anticholinergic side effects like dry mouth, constipation, and urinary retention are common, especially in older adults.

- They are not recommended for long-term use or for treating chronic insomnia.

Abuse and misuse of 'sleep aids'
The abuse and misuse of OTC 'sleep aids' depicted in this story is a real problem.

Here are some relevant UK and US links:

NICE guidelines (for short-term insomnia) in the United Kingdom explicitly state *"do not recommend OTC sleep aids"*.

https://cks.nice.org.uk/topics/insomnia/managemen
t/managing-insomnia/#short-term-insomnia-less-3-
months

United Kingdom's General Pharmaceutical Council
"spotlight" on cyclizine:
https://www.pharmacyregulation.org/about-us/news-
and-updates/regulate/patient-safety-spotlight-risks-
cyclizine-misuse-and-promoting-safe-provision-
patients

Antihistamine-related deaths in England: Are the high
safety profiles of antihistamines leading to their unsafe
use?
https://bpspubs.onlinelibrary.wiley.com/doi/full/10.
1111/bcp.14819

National Library of Medicine. (2022). Doxylamine:
MedlinePlus Drug Information. Available at:
https://medlineplus.gov/druginfo/meds/a682537.ht
ml

Mayo Clinic (2021). Sleep aids: Understand over-the-
counter options. Available at:
https://www.mayoclinic.org/healthy-lifestyle/adult-
health/in-depth/sleep-aids/art-20047860

www.ingramcontent.com/pod-product-compliance
Lightning Source LLC
Chambersburg PA
CBHW050950050726

47592CB00007B/2507